"OH FOR SMART"®

Other Books
By
Sven Olsen

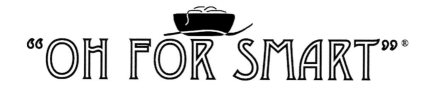

"OH FOR SMART"®

THE NORTHERN MINNESOTA PRETTY GOOD WAY TO LOSE WEIGHT AND GET IN SHAPE

by
Sven Olsen

Illustrations and Photographs
by
An A, Three Bs, and a D

Published by
DMcD Productions, Inc.
Grand Rapids, Minnesota

POSSIBLE REVIEWS
THAT HAVE NOT BEEN WRITTEN YET

"This book says it all."
-The Rainy Lake Recorder

"All… that needs to be said is right here."
-The New York Times

"Olsen has been there and back. It is so refreshing to finally read
an honest account of something a lot of us
are trying to come to terms with."
-The Washington Post

"A complicated tale told by a master."
-The Los Angeles Times

"There are a lot of books about health, nutrition, and fitness.
This one is in a league of its own."
-Journal of Scientific Charts

"A must read."
-NBC, ABC, CBS, CNN

"Better than any of Olsen's other books."
-The Bovey Bulletin

"I'd love to get him on my show."
-Oprah

"Only after he's been on mine."
-Jay Leno

"Don't forget NPR."
-National Public Radio

iv

NOTICE

This book provides a detailed method
to lose weight and get in shape.

If you have any health issues, please consult your physician
before starting the "OH FOR SMART" routine.

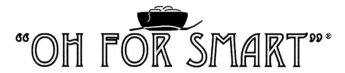

"OH FOR SMART"®

THE NORTHERN MINNESOTA PRETTY GOOD WAY
TO LOSE WEIGHT AND GET IN SHAPE

For more information please contact
www.ohforsmart.com

Cover design, illustrations, and photographs
by
An A, Three Bs, and a D

Library of Congress Control Number: 2005932459

ISBN 0-9771521-0-3
ISBN 978-0-977-15210-0

SAN: 256-9019

To Hilwa,
who is a good dog.

TESTIMONIALS

""OH FOR SMART"" changed my life, for the better, I mean."
-Barb Olsen
Warba, Minnesota

"What I like about "OH FOR SMART" is that it makes you think about other stuff while you lose weight and get in shape."
-Phil Olsen
Portland, Oregon

"Guess what word you NEVER see in "OH FOR SMART"?
It's a four-letter word that starts with 'd' and
ends with 't' and has two vowels in the middle.
You can't find it, the "d" word, not once. Go figure."
-Margaret Olsen-Johnson
Bethesda, Maryland

"I burned a bunch of calories just turning the pages."
-Dan Olsen
Bernardston, Massachusetts

"I sent a few copies of the book to my friends and relatives because they're all overweight and out of shape, you know, slobs."
-Jimmy Olsen
Voorheesville, New York

"I liked the list, recipe, suggestions, and scientific-looking chart."
-Harper Olsen
Wilmington, North Carolina

"When are they going to make the "OH FOR SMART" movie?"
-Haley Olsen
Fairplay, Colorado

PREFACE

Two, maybe three years ago, I woke up and said,
"Sven, you should lose some weight and get in shape."
So I did.
I wrote this book, too.

Sven Olsen

"OH FOR SMART"®

THE NORTHERN MINNESOTA
PRETTY GOOD WAY
TO LOSE WEIGHT
AND
GET IN SHAPE

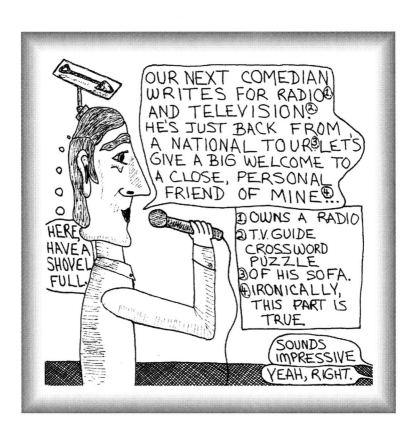

CONTENTS

NOTICE	v
TESTIMONIALS	viii
PREFACE	ix
CHAPTER ONE	1
CHAPTER TWO	5
ANOTHER NOTICE	9
CHAPTER THREE	11
CHAPTER FOUR	15
CHAPTER FIVE	19
CHAPTER SIX	23
CHAPTER SEVEN	27
NEW NOTICE	31
CHAPTER EIGHT	33
CHAPTER NINE	37
ONE MORE NOTICE	41
CHAPTER TEN	43
CHAPTER ELEVEN	51
CHAPTER TWELVE	59
CHAPTER THIRTEEN	67
BONUS NOTICE	71
CHAPTER FOURTEEN	73
CHAPTER FIFTEEN	77
CHAPTER SIXTEEN	81
CHAPTER SEVENTEEN	85
CONCLUSION	89
LAST NOTICE	93
APPENDIX A	95
APPENDIX B	97
APPENDIX C	99

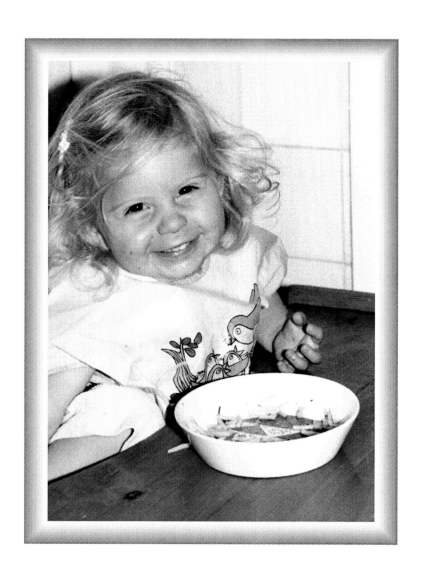

CHAPTER
ONE

1

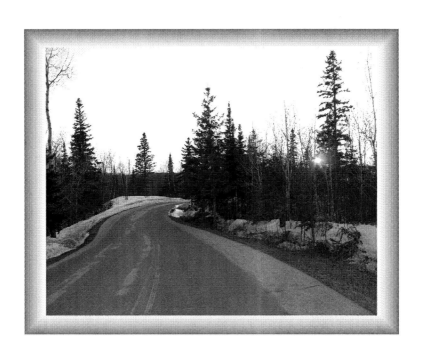

If you are overweight,
eat less.

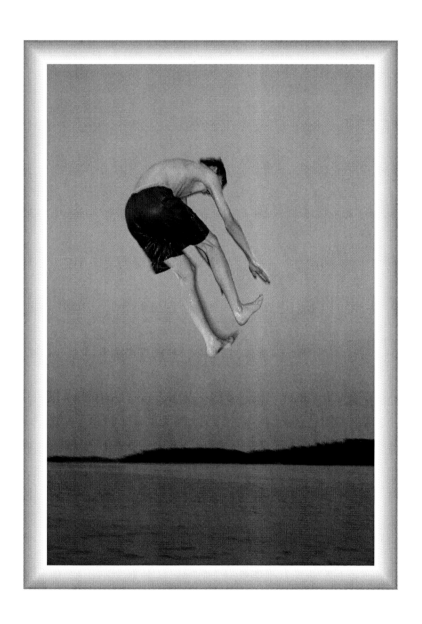

CHAPTER TWO

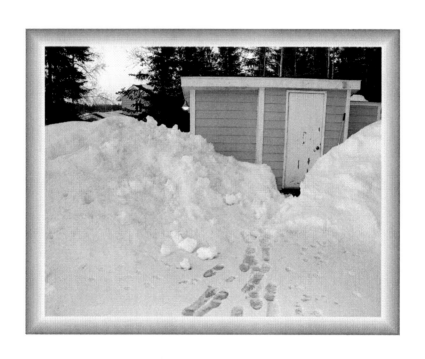

If you are out of shape,
exercise more.

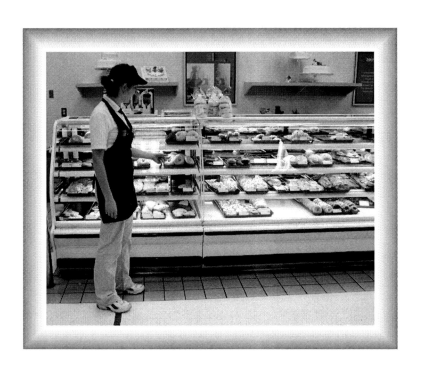

ANOTHER NOTICE

That is pretty much it.
But my wife told me that if people are going to buy a book,
it has to have lots of chapters.
So I have some more chapters after this.
They are full of things that anybody
could figure out by themselves.
The important stuff is in Chapter One and Chapter Two.

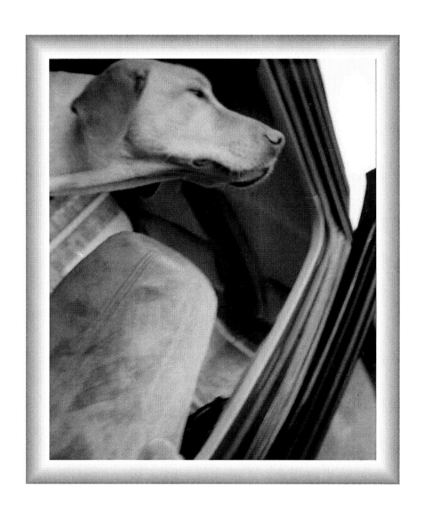

CHAPTER THREE

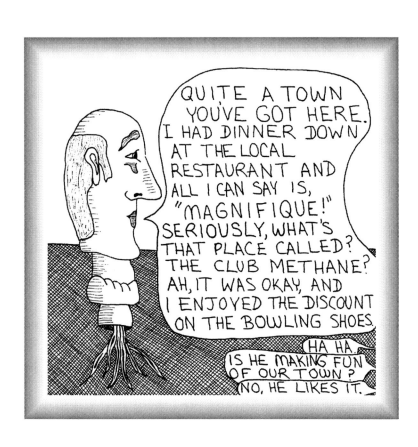

12

For a few months,
do what it is says in Chapter One and Chapter Two.

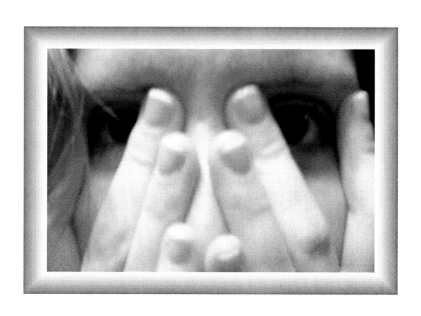

CHAPTER
FOUR

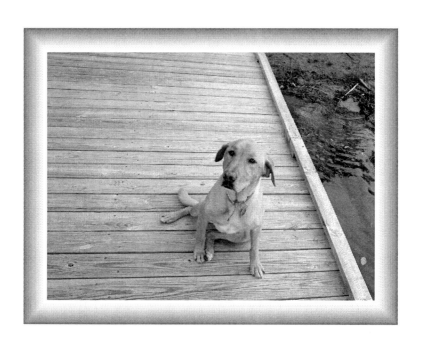

If you are losing weight and getting in shape,
keep doing what it says in Chapter One and Chapter Two.

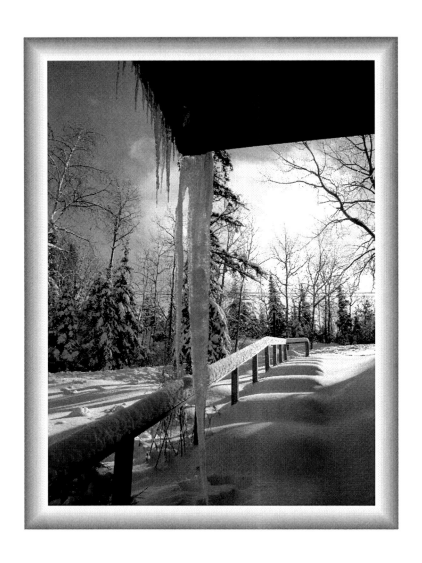

CHAPTER
FIVE

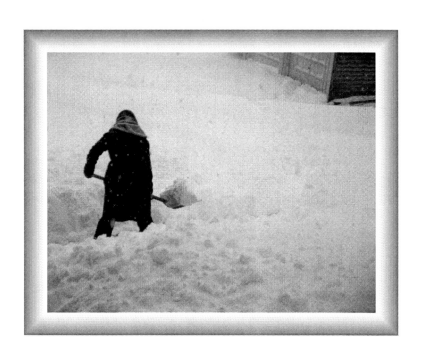

After a few months,
if you are not losing weight and not getting in shape,
go back and do more of what it says
in Chapter One and Chapter Two.

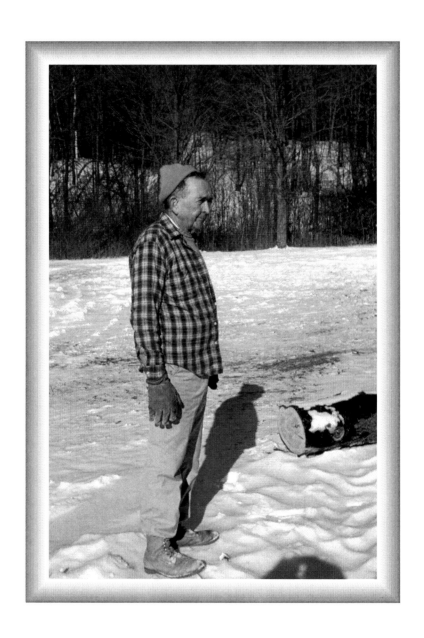

CHAPTER SIX

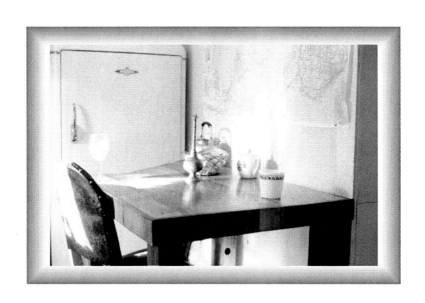

Don't get carried away with just doing the part in Chapter One
about eating less
and not doing the part in Chapter Two
about exercising more.
Eating less while sitting on a couch
is kind of like fishing without a hook…
it is going to be real tough to catch anything.

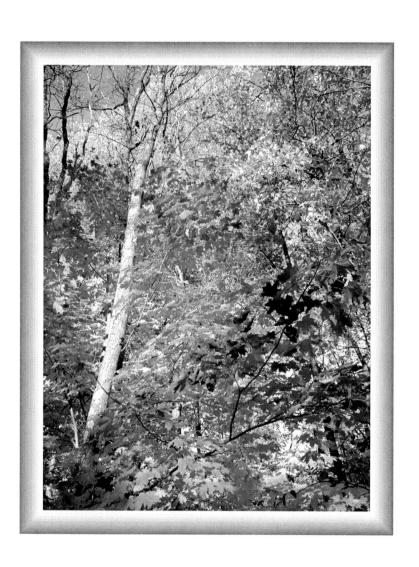

CHAPTER SEVEN

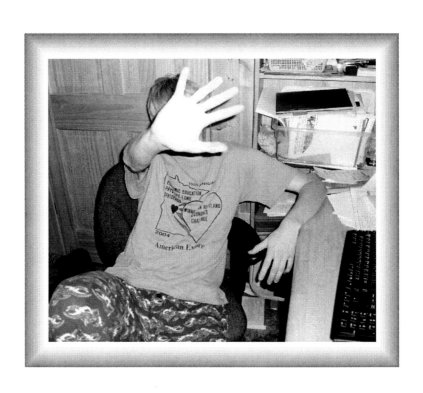

28

Same goes for the other way around.

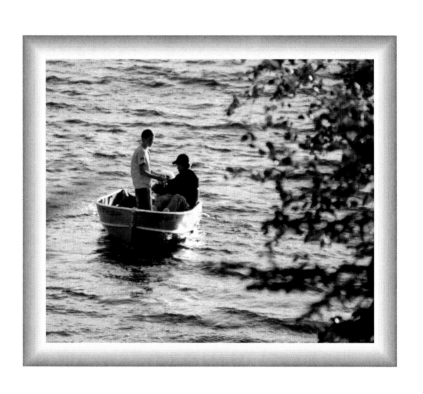

NEW NOTICE

I have been informed that I should be more specific.

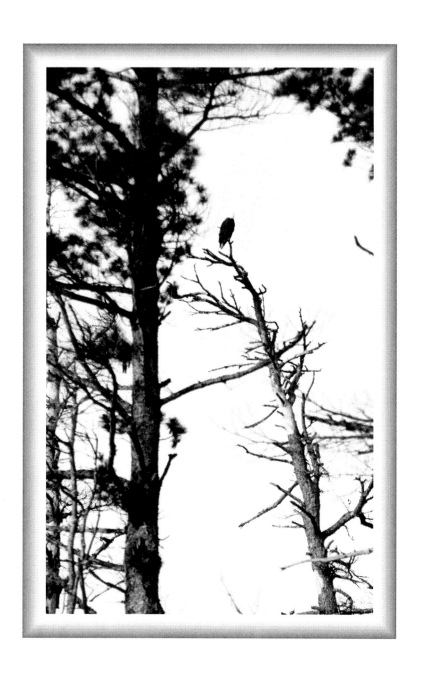

CHAPTER EIGHT

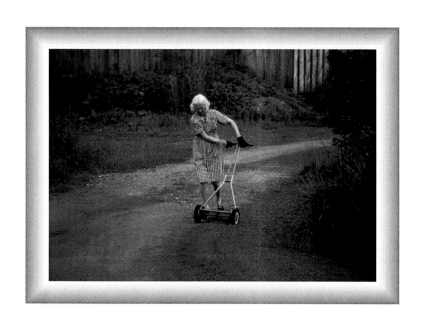

Don't get carried away with just doing the part in Chapter Two
about exercising more
and not doing the part in Chapter One
about eating less.
Chowing down after going for a walk
is kind of like fishing without a line…
you are going through the motions,
but you are not going to catch any fish.

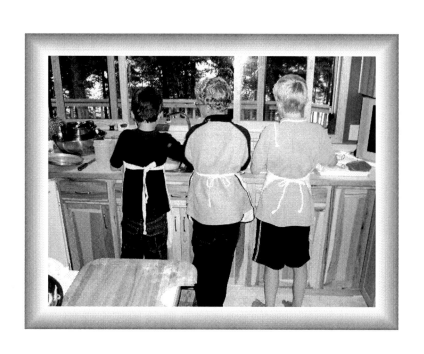

CHAPTER NINE

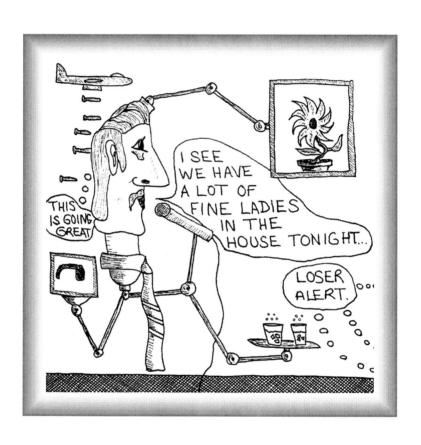

38

After a while,
if you find that you are
losing weight and getting in shape,
then you know you have found the right balance
for doing what it says in Chapter One and Chapter Two.
Then you can start thinking about eating right,
you know the stuff they teach in Health class.

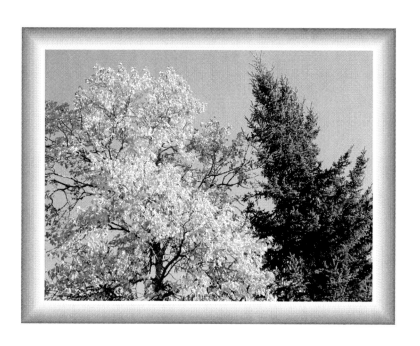

ONE MORE NOTICE

My daughter tells me when it comes to
losing weight and getting in shape,
people like to read lists and recipes and
suggestions and scientific-looking charts.
I said OK, let's include a list, a recipe, a few suggestions,
and a scientific-looking chart.

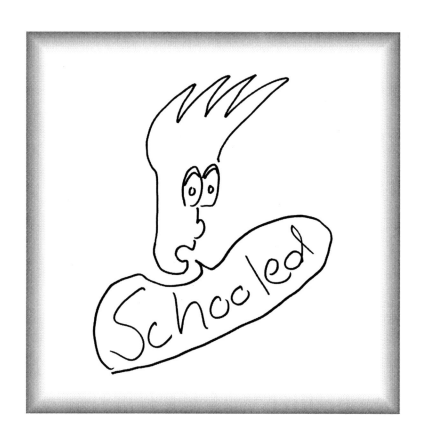

CHAPTER TEN

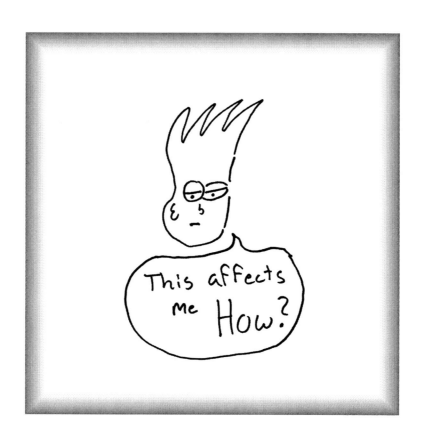

A LIST OF BOOKS AND MAGAZINES

I asked some friends if they had any books or magazines
that said pretty much the same thing
as what I am saying in this "OH FOR SMART" book.
They said yes.
So here is a list of books and magazines.
My neighbor two houses down is a lawyer and she says that
I should make it clear that by listing these books and magazines
it does not mean I think they are good
or that you should do what they say.
I don't know most of them.
Some I know are good.
I can tell you that the first two are great.

45

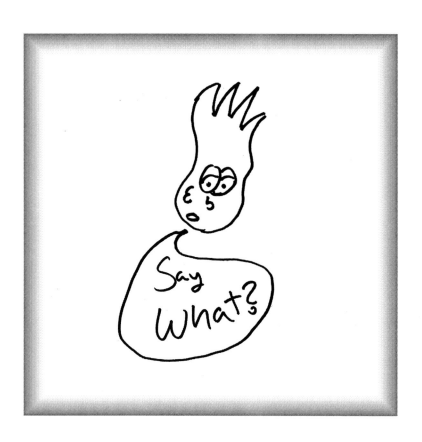

A LIST OF
BOOKS AND MAGAZINES

National Geographic August 2004, *Stretching* (Bob Anderson and illustrated by Jean Anderson), *The Way To Eat* (David L. Katz), *The Pathway* (Laurel Mellin), *The McDougall Program for Maximum Weight Loss* (John McDougall), *Eat More,Weigh Less* (Dean Ornish), *Dr. Shapiro's Picture Perfect Weight Loss* (Howard M. Shapiro), *Eating Well for Optimum Health* (Andrew Weil), *Dieting for Dummies* (Jane Kirby), *The Soy Zone* (Barry Sears), *Weight Watchers: New Complete Cookbook* (Weight Watchers), *Body for Life* (Bill Phillips), *Sugar Busters!* (H. Leighton Steward), *Dr. Atkins' New Diet Revolution* (Robert Atkins), *The Carbohydrate Addict's Lifespan Program* (Richard Heller), *Fit For Life* (Harvey Diamond), *4 Blood Types, 4 Diets, Eat Right 4 Your Type* (Peter J. D'Adamo), *The Tibetan Book of Living and Dying* (Sogyal Rinpoche), *Cancer and Nutrition* (Charles B. Simone), *Plato Not Prozac* (Lou Marinoff), *The Arthritis Foundation's Guide To Alternative Therapies* (Judith Horstman), *Total Health Makeover* (Marilu Henner), *Western Academy of Beijing International Cookbook* (WAB PTA), *The Conscience of a Liberal* (Paul Wellstone), *Healing Mind, Healthy Woman* (Alice Domar), *Living Low-Carb* (Fran McCullough), *The Wisdom of Menopause* (Christiane Northrup), *Natural Family Doctor* (Andrew Stanway), *Cooking Light Magazine*, *The Road Less Traveled* (M. Scott Peck), *Heavenly Delights* (St. Joseph's Parish, Grand Rapids), *New Cook Book* (Better Homes and Gardens), *All Class Reunion Cookbook 2000* (Falls High School), *Home Style Korean Cooking in Pictures* (Cho Joong Ok), *Egyptian Cuisine* (Nagwa E. Khalil), *Arabian Cuisine* (Anne Marie Weiss-Armush), *Family Favorites Volume I and II* (Dhahran Women's Group), *Rodale's Basic Natural Foods Cookbook* (Charles Gerras), *Recipes From Our Friends* (Itasca County Family YMCA), *Untitled and Other Poems* (Lee Norton), *Joy of Cooking* (Irma S. Rombauer), *Eater's Choice* (Ron Goor), *Nutrition Book* (Jane Brody), *Favorite Recipes From The Warm Hearts of the Icebox* (International Falls Elks), *Couscous and Other Good Food From Morocco* (Paula Wolfert), *Feed Me* (Harper Dircks), *Great Good Food, Lucious Lower-Fat Cooking* (Julee Rosso), *Tax Implications of A Healthy Lifestyle* (William Gruen), *The Glycemic Index* (Rick Gallop), *The Birmingham Idea* (Alana Helms), *The Maker's Table* (Jibreel and Gideon Powell), *The South Beach Diet* (Arthur Agatston), *The Ultimate Weight Solution* (Phil McGraw), *The Zone: A Dietary Road Map* (Barry Sears), *Protein Power* (Michael R. Eades), *Dieting with the Duchess* (Sarah, Duchess of York), *Volume Versus Density: Engineering A Healthy Diet* (Ronald and William Helms), *Pilates Workbook: Illustrated Step-By-Step Guide to Matwork Techniques* (Michael King), *Pilates for Wimps* (Jennifer DeLuca), *The Guitar and Tambourine Exercise Routine* (Billy McDonald), *Diet Trials* (Lyndel Costain), *The 9 Truths About Weight Loss* (Daniel S. Kirschenbaum), *Menopause without Weight Gain* (Debra Waterhouse), *The Vegetarian Sports Nutrition Guide* (Lisa Dorfman), *ACSM Fitness Book* (the American College of Sports Medicine), *A Study of Science Fiction Food* (Donald Renquist), *Precision Heart Rate Training* (Edmund R. Burke), *Fit for Two: The Official YMCA Prenatal Exercise Guide* (YMCA of the USA), *The Complete Guide to Postnatal Fitness: The Official Central YMCA Guide* (Judy DiFiore), *The New Encyclopedia of Modern Bodybuilding* (Arnold Schwarzenegger), *Strength Training Anatomy* (Frédéric Delavier), *The Art of Expressing the Human Body* (Bruce Lee, John Little), *When Working Out Isn't Working Out: A Mind/Body Guide to Conquering UnidentifiedFitness Obstacles* (Michael Gerrish), *No Thanks, We'll Take A Canoe: Adventures on Rainy Lake* (Arnie and Maxine Long), *Health Fitness Instructor's Handbook* (Edward T. Howley and B. Don Franks), *ACSM's Exercise Management for Persons with Chronic Diseases and Disabilities* (J. Larry Durstine and Geoffrey E. Moore), *Exercise for Older Adults* (Richard T. Cotton*), The Pritikin Principle* (Robert Pritikin), *Choose to Lose* (Ron Goor), *Eat, Drink, and Be Healthy: The Harvard Medical School Guide to Healthy Eating* (Walter C. Willett), *Ruthless Democracy* (Timothy B. Powell), *The Perricone Promise* (Nicholas Perricone), *The Mediterranean Diet* (Marissa Cloutier), *Closing the Deal Down Under* (Andrew Crisp), *The Culprit and the Cure* (Steven G. Aldana), *Banish Your Belly* (Kenton Robinson), *I Get It* (Emma Bole), *The Men's Health Guide to Peak Conditioning* (Richard Laliberte*), Play Hard - Get Strong* (Andrew Helms), *The Cabana Lifestyle* (Dave Gruen), *Walking with Your Horse* (Kirsten Harris), *Golf Myths About Exercise* (David and Jack Powell), *The Mind Body Workout With Pilates and The Alexander Technique* (Lynne Robinson), *Affirmative and Negative: The Debate Over Salt, Butter and Popcorn* (Brian McDonald), *The Art of Swimming Fast* (Sally Powell), *Horsemanship and The Alexander Experience* (Daniel Pevsner), *Health Maintenance Through Food and Nutrition* (Helen D. Ullrich), *Food and Nutrition Information Guide* (Paula Szilard), *World Food Problem: A Selective Bibliography of Reviews* (Miloslav Rechcigl), *How To Stay Trim and Still Play Poker All Night* (Amjad Ghori), *Natural Foods: Nutritional Value a Bibliography* (Petro Berrange), *Nutrition and Aging: A Selected Bibliography* (Barbara Elaine St. Clair), *Ten Easy Stretches Before Deer Hunting* (Jennifer Prettyman Butterfield), *Nutritional Value of Indigenous Wild Plants* (Joel Elias), *International Cultural and Commercial Approaches to Eating Right* (Michael and Martha Keaveny), *Food And Paradise* (Dietrich Gruen), *Food and Nutrition in the Middle East 1970-1986* (Gail Harrison), *A Veritable Scoff* (Maura Hanrahan), *A Different Shade of Colonialism: Egypt, Great Britain, and the Mastery of the Sudan* (Eve Troutt Powell), *Abs Diet* (David Zinczenko), *Healthy Fashion; Fashionable Health* (Madeline Gruen), *South Beach Diet Cookbook* (Arthur S. Agatston), *Understanding Nutrition With Infotrac* (Eleanor Noss Whitney), *How To Compete Legally and Safely Against Your Brother in Cross Country* (Will and Sam Jevne), *The Men's Health Cover Model Workout* (Owen McKibbin), *Counterfeiting Exposed: How to Protect Your Brand and Market Share* (Mark Turnage), *Ask A Dietitian, Ask a Librarian, Ask Me,* (Mary McDonald), *Walleye Wonders* (Jimmy Nelson, Nolan Kerr and Luke Kelberer), *A Beach Bum's Daily Exercise Routine* (Allen Renquist), *Sure Lightens The Place Up* (Steve King and Mike Heibel), *Shore Lunch* (Michael Currin), *Natural Healthy World* (Greta Swanson), *How To Do The Bus Stop and Other Great Dances* (Art Kelberer), *Five Easy Ways to Pick the Right Bait* (Ben Currin), *Yoga The Spirit And Practice of Moving Into Stillness,* (Erich Schiffmann), *Structural Yoga Therapy* (Mukunda Stiles), *Yoga The Iyengar Way* (Mira Silva and Shyam Mehta), *We Are Men: Camping in the American and Canadian Rockies* (Mark and Eric Gruen), *Yoga for Wellness* (Gary Kraftsow), *The Heart Of Yoga* (TKV Desikachar), *Awakening The Spine* (Vanda Scaravelli), *Surfing Strategies to Stay Slim* (Will Burgess), *Yoga A Gem For Women* (Geeta S. Iyengar), *The Complete Illustrated Book Of Yoga* (Swami Vishnu-devananda), *Basketball for Life* (Simon Kerr), *Integral Yoga Hatha* (Swami Satchidananda), *The Breathing Book* (Donna Farhi), *Structural Yoga Therapy* (Mukunda Stiles), *Pizza, Sausage and Bacon: How To Play Soccer* (Philip McDonald and Carter Rohling), *Yoga For Wellness* (Gary Kraftsow), *Back Care Basics* (Mary Pullig Schatz), *Relax and Renew* (Judith Lasatar), *Preparing For Birth With Yoga* (Janet Balaskas), *Miracles Happen and Other Great Bedtime Stories* (Nathan Pearson and Simon Long), *Cheering For Health, Volume One* (Chessie Gruen), *Danish Talking Exercises* (Morten and Mads), *You Don't Know What You've Got Until It's Gone, So Get Rid of It As Soon As Possible* (Zanube Thababaru), *Tennis Under A Noon Day Sun* (Ricky "Duke" Snyder), *A Child's Garden of Yoga* (Baba Hari Dass), *Yoga For Children* (Mary Stewart), *Like A Fish In Water* (Isabelle Koch), *Swimming From South Jackfish to Chapel Hill* (Tina Renquist),

47

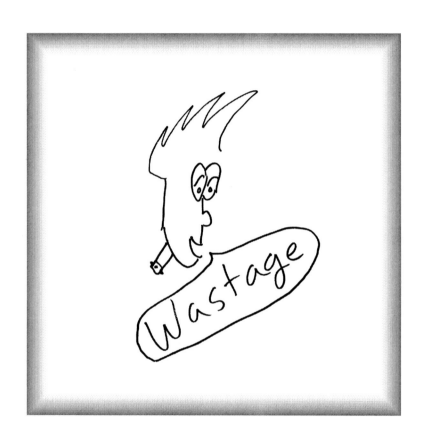

A LIST OF
BOOKS AND MAGAZINES

Wheels of Life - A User's Guide To The Chakra System (Anodea Judith), *Kundalini Yoga For Body, Mind and Beyond* (Ravi Singh), *Full Catastrophe Living* (Jon Kabat-Zinn), *Technology as a Determining Factor in Television News Coverage: A Case Study of NBC News Cairo from 1973 to 1985* (David McDonald), *Wherever You Go, There You Are* (Jon Kabat-Zinn), *When Things Fall Apart* (Pema Chodron), *A Path With Heart* (Jack Kornfield), *Woman Awake: A Celebration of Women's Wisdom* (Christina Feldman), *Women Of Wisdom* (Tsultrim Allione), *Insight Meditation - The Practice Of Freedom* (Joseph Goldstein), *Peace Is Every Step* (Thich Nhat Hanh), *Being Peace* (Thich Nhat Hanh), *The Miracle of Mindfulness* (Thich Nhat Hanh), *Vipassana Meditation as Taught By S.N. Goenka* (William Hart), *Be Here Now* (Ram Dass), *Body for Life* (Bill Phillips), *The Men's Health Hard Body Plan: The Ultimate 12-Week Program for Burning Fat and Building Muscle: Featuring the Hard-Body Diet and the Revolutionary New Quick-Set Path to Power* (Larry Keller), *The Complete Guide to Walking for Health, Weight Loss, and Fitness* (Mark Fenton), *Get Stronger by Stretching With Thera-Band* (Noa Spector-Flock), *Relax into Stretch: Instant Flexiblity Through Mastering Muscle Tension* (Pavel Tsatsouline), *Bullet-Proof Abs: The Second Edition of Beyond Crunches* (Pavel Tsatsouline), *Weight Training: Steps to Success* (Thomas R. Baechle), *Lacrosse Is It* (TJ Powell), *Power to the People!: Russian Strength Training Secrets for Every American* (Pavel Tsatsouline), *Buff Brides: The Complete Guide to Getting Shape and Looking Great for Your Wedding Day* (Sue Fleming), *The Mountain Biker's Training Bible: A Complete Training Guide for the Competitive Mountain Biker* (Joe Friel), *Max Contraction Training: The Scientifically Proven Program for Building Muscle Mass in Minimum Time* (John Little), *Exercise After Pregnancy:* (Helene Byrne), *Be a Loser!: Lose Inches Fast--No Diet* (Greer Childers), *Pilates Powerhouse* (Mari Winsor), *Women Han Nu Li, Women Jiao Ban, Every Night It's On My Mind* (Ma Shanling), *The Pilates Body: The Ultimate At-Home Guide to Strengthening, Lengthening, and Toning Your Body--Without Machines* (Brooke Siler), *Abs on the Ball: A Pilates Approach to Building Superb Abdominals* (Colleen Craig), *The Pilates Workout Journal: An Exercise Diary and Conditioning Guide* (Mari Winsor), *Osteopilates: Increase Bone Density Reduce Fracture Risk Look and Feel Great* (Karena Thek Lineback*), Yogilates: Integrating Yoga and Pilates for Complete Fitness, Strength, and Flexibility* (Jonathan Urla), *Pilates' Return to Life Through Contrology* (Joseph H. Pilates), *Royal Canadian Air Force Exercises* (Bull Winkle), *The Little Pilates Book* (Erika Dillman), *Pilates on the Ball: The World's Most Popular Workout Using the Exercise Ball* (Colleen Craig), *Football, Soccer, Baseball... Whatever! Let's Just Play* (Jeffrey Gruen), *Pilates for Dummies* (Ellie Herman), *Pilates for Beginners* (Kelline Stewart), *Pilates for Pregnancy: Gentle and Effective Techniques for Before and After Birth* (Anna Selby), *Jennifer Kries' Pilates Plus Method: The Unique Combination of Yoga, Dance, and Pilates* (Jennifer Kries), *Pilates: Body in Motion* (Alycea Ungaro), *The Pilates Edge: An Athelete's Guide to Strength and Performance* (Karrie Adamany), *The Nutrition Reporter, Wellspring Newsletter, How To Make Your Wake Boarding Fantasies Become Reality* (Robert Renquist), *Food for Life Newsletter, Japanese and Egyptian Eating Utensils* (Jennifer Renquist), *Vegetarian & Natural Health, Burn Calories in a Marching Band* (Katie Helms), *When The Band Stops Playing* (Jake Kelberer), *Veggie Life Magazine, Healthy Weight Journal, Weight Watchers News, Diabetes Forecast, Diabetic Cooking, Eating Well, Fit Pregnancy, Fitness, Out Fishing* (John Renquist), *Herb Companion, Herbs for Health, Life Extension, LowCarb Energy, LowCarb Living, Men's Health, Natural Health, Nutrition Health Review, Who Is Winning If the Score Is Tied?* (Angie Liedke*), The Concise History of the Queen Mary* (Margaret Kelberer), *Looking Good On The Lake* (Haley Nelson, Gracie Kerr, Vicky Kelberer), *DASH* (Krissy Currin), *Tools To Eat Well* (Graham Dircks), *Muscle Elegance, Muscle Media, MuscleMag, Muscular Development, Looking Better On The Lake* (Sophie Currin and Avery Kerr), *Natural Bodybuilding, Natural Muscle, NPC News, Oxygen Fitness, Physical, Planet, PowerMag, The Merck Manual of Medical Information: Home Edition* (Robert Berkow), *Discovering Nutrition* (Paul Insel, Don Ross and R. Elaine Turner), *Effective Protest Signs in the Deep South* (Eileen Helms), *Dieting for Dummies* (Jane Kirby), *Monthly Nutrition Companion: 31 Ways to a Healthier Lifestyle* (Paul Insel, Don Ross and R. Elaine Turner), *Snacking Habits for Healthy Living* (The American Dietetic Association), *Diet Simple* (Katherine Tallmadge), *Eating Well on Campus* (Ann Selkowitz Litt), *The Essential Guide to Nutrition and the Foods We Eat* (The American Dietetic Association with Jean Pennington), *Minerals, Supplements & Vitamins: the Essential Guide* (H. Winter Griffith), *The New Nutrition* (Felicia Busch), *Nutrition Concepts and Controversies, Eighth Edition* (Frances Sizer and Eleanor Whitney), *Portion Savvy: The 30-Day Smart Plan for Eating Well* (Carrie Latt Wiatt and Elizabeth Miles), *Stealth Health: How to Sneak Nutrition Painlessly into Your Diet* (Evelyn Tribole), *Super Nutrition After 50* (Densie Webb and Elizabeth Ward), *Your Personality Prescription: Optimal Health Through Personality Profiling* (Roberta Schwartz Wennik), *Intolerance Nutrition Guide* (Merri Lou Dobler), *The Gluten-Free Gourmet: Living Well Without Wheat* (Bette Hagman), *Kids with Celiac Disease* (Danna Korn), *Prop Repair* (Mark Levene), *The New Family Cookbook for People with Diabetes* (The American Dietetic Association and the American Diabetes Association), *The Philosophy Behind Computer Games* (Daniel McDonald), *The American Diabetes Association Guide to Healthy Restaurant Eating* (Hope Warshaw), *The Diabetes Carbohydrate and Fat Gram Guide* (Lea Ann Holzmeister), *The Diabetes Food & Nutrition Bible: A Complete Guide to Planning, Shopping, Cooking, and Eating* (Hope Warshaw and Robyn Webb), *Month of Meals: Classic Cooking -- Quick & Easy Menus for People With Diabetes* (The American Diabetes Association), *No-Fuss Diabetes Recipes for 1 or 2* (Jackie Boucher, Marcia Hayes and Jane Stephenson), *Complete Guide to Sports Nutrition* (Monique Ryan), *Endurance Sports Nutrition* (Suzanne Girand Eberle), *Nancy Clark's Food Guide for Marathoners* (Nancy Clark), *Power Eating: Build Muscle Boost Energy Cut Fat, Second Edition* (Susan Kleiner and Maggie Greenwood-Robinson), *Food Folklore: Tales and Truths About What We Eat* (Roberta L. Duyff), *Bowes and Church's Food Values of Portions Commonly Used* (Jean Pennington), *Latin for Health* (Jane Macartney), *The Complete Book of Food Counts* (Corrine T. Netzer), *Herbs of Choice: The Therapeutic Use of Phytomedicinals* (Varro E. Tyler), *The New Food Lover's Tiptionary* (Sharon Tyler Herbst), *Wellness Foods A to Z* (Sheldon Margen and editors of UC Berkeley Wellness Letter), *What Einstein Told His Cook* (Robert L. Wolke), *If Your Child Is Overweight: A Guide for Parents, Second Edition* (Susan Kosharek), *ADA Guide to Healthy Eating for Kids: How Your Children Can Eat Smart from 5 to 12* (The American Dietetic Association), *Roof* (Mumchick), *Pregnancy Nutrition: Good Health for You and Your Baby* (The American Dietetic Association), *American Academy of Pediatrics Guide to Your Child's Nutrition* (William H. Dietz and Loraine Stern), *Vaulting to Health* (Brian McDonald), *Child of Mine: Feeding With Love and Good Sense* (Ellyn Satter), *Eating Expectantly* (Bridget Swinney), *Food Fight: A Guide to Eating Disorders for Preteens and Their Parents* (Janet Bode), *Food, Fun n' Fitness: Designing Healthy Lifestyles for Our Children* (Mary Friesz), *Food Rules!* (Bill Haduch, Rick Stromoski and Lisa Moore), *Healthy Foods, Healthy Kids* (Elizabeth Ward), *The Nursing Mother's Companion* (Kathleen Huggins), *Raising Happy, Healthy, Weight-wise Kids* (Judy Toews and Nicole Parton), *When You're Expecting Twins, Triplets or Quads: A Complete Resource* (Barbara Luke and Tamara Eberlein), *The WEEK.*

49

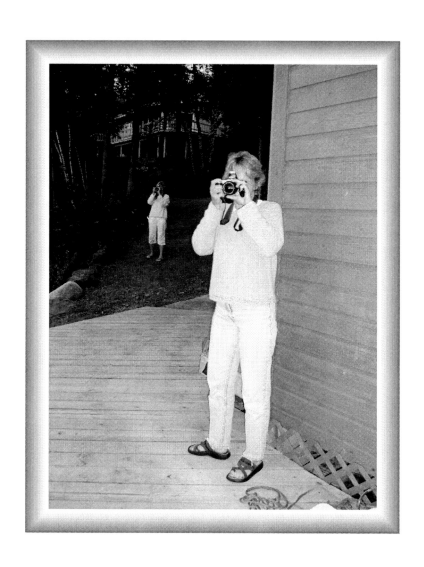

CHAPTER ELEVEN

A RECIPE FOR FRIDAY NIGHT SPAGHETTI

Every Friday night I make spaghetti.
It is sort of a family tradition.
My kids don't always eat the sauce.
They just like spaghetti with cheese on top.
I don't think I know anyone
who doesn't know how to make spaghetti.
This is how I make it.
It feeds about two to six people for about two to four days
depending on how many teenagers pass through the house.

A RECIPE FOR
FRIDAY NIGHT SPAGHETTI

1.) You fill a big pot with water. Not to the top but more than halfway. Put it on the hottest burner. Splash some oil in the water. Don't add salt to the water. That is not necessary because there is too much salt in food these days.

2.) Get another pot, not so big. Brown one or two pounds of meat in it. It could be burger, pork, sausage, or whatever.

3.) Add some spices to the burger. I add the green ones like Italian or oregano. I also add lemon pepper because I like lemon. Don't add spices to pork or sausage. They already have enough. Don't add salt to anything. That is not necessary because there is too much salt in food these days. I sometimes splash on some soy sauce but only on burger because soy sauce has a lot of salt in it.

4.) After the ground meat is brown, dump out any grease that is left in the pot. If you pour it down the sink, you are only going to have a problem with the plumbing later on.

5.) Put in one can of diced tomatoes. Use diced because the cans with wholes tomatoes or stewed tomatoes have big pieces which the kids don't like as much. Diced is the way to go. I use the kind that says "NO SALT" on the label because there is too much salt in food these days. But sometimes I use the kind that says "ITALIAN SEASONING" on the label if it is on sale.

6.) Let the meat and the diced tomatoes get to know each other in the pot. I sometimes add mushrooms now, but then I know the kids are not going to eat the sauce.

7.) By now the water is starting to think about boiling. I hope you put a cover on the water pot because that makes the water start to boil faster.

A RECIPE FOR
FRIDAY NIGHT SPAGHETTI

8.) Turn on the oven to around 300 degrees.

9.) Right around now is when you have to stay in the kitchen for about 15 minutes otherwise something will go wrong. So if there is a game on in another room, turn up the volume.

10.) Add a big jar of spaghetti sauce to the ground meat and diced tomatoes. You can do a taste test with all the different kinds. I use Prego Traditional. Stay away from the other kinds with onions, meat, sausage or whatever. You can also experiment with some of those fancy ones in the smaller jars that cost more, but be prepared for the kids not to like it. I use some of Paul Newman's sauces because he gives money to charity but I can't say that his sauces are my favorites. I stay away from any sauce that has cheese in it. How can that stuff stay fresh sitting on a shelf for weeks.

11.) Don't add salt or more spices because there are plenty of both in whatever jar you get. Besides, there is too much salt in food these days.

12.) Stir the sauce and watch out that the flame is not so high that the sauce explodes like a volcano and splatters all over the stove and the counter and the dishes and the cabinets. If it does, wipe it up right away otherwise it will get hard and you are only going to have a problem later.

13.) Right after you have added the big jar of sauce and stirred it a bit, the water should be boiling. You are about ten minutes away from the finish line. Put some of that good bread that you have to bake before you eat into the oven for about ten minutes. If you want, you can slap some butter and garlic powder on it to make garlic bread.

A RECIPE FOR
FRIDAY NIGHT SPAGHETTI

14.) When the bread is in the oven, then you put a box of thin spaghetti into the boiling water. Do not get regular spaghetti or fettuccini or any other kind except maybe elbow macaroni. All those other kinds are just more pasta that fill you up. Angel Hair is OK if you are in a rush because it takes only about five minutes to cook. But Angel Hair starts clumping together after a while and does not taste as good the next day. With thin spaghetti it makes you think like you are eating more and you can put on more sauce. Deciding whether to cook one pound or two pounds of spaghetti depends on how many teenagers are in the house. Always cook too much spaghetti. Always use the whole box. Always have leftovers for lunch the next day.

15.) Now you are stirring the spaghetti and stirring the sauce, so you can't leave the kitchen to watch the game unless there is a really big play. But you better hurry back or you are only going to have a problem later.

16.) When the spaghetti is ready, everything is ready and that is when you can turn off the two burners and the oven. Forget about the test of seeing if the spaghetti is ready by throwing it onto the ceiling to see if it sticks. That test doesn't work because the spaghetti will stick before it is fully cooked. The way to tell if the spaghetti is ready is to take a few pieces, let them cool in the strainer thing in the sink (did I mention that you should put the strainer thing in the sink?), and then taste it. When the spaghetti is bendy but not too stiff and not too squooshy, then it is ready. The Italians call it "al dente". You can look that up on the internet. It means "to the teeth" like dental or dentist. The Italians know what they are talking about when it comes to pasta.

A RECIPE FOR
FRIDAY NIGHT SPAGHETTI

17.) Turn the cold water on so that it goes next to the strainer thing not in it. The spaghetti pot is hot (duh) so use a towel or those big mittens to pick it up and pour everything into the strainer thing. The cold water is just to mix with the boiling hot water as it goes down the drain. Don't run the cold water on the spaghetti. That just cools down the spaghetti. Hot spaghetti is better than cold spaghetti.

18.) Put a little water in the bottom of the empty big pot so that any leftover spaghetti stuff does not get sticky and hard to clean.

19.) After the water has drained out of the strainer thing, dump all the spaghetti into a big bowl that is sitting on one of those things that protects the counter from hot dishes.

20.) Spray water over the empty strainer thing so that any leftover spaghetti stuff does not get sticky and hard to clean.

21.) Pour lots of olive oil onto the spaghetti and stir it. Use Extra Virgin olive oil because that tastes better than the other kind. Your kids will let you know if you have poured too much olive oil onto the spaghetti.

22.) Take the bread out of the oven with a towel or those big mittens (duh).

23.) Check that the oven and the burners are all off. Get a damp rag and clean up any mess now because if you wait until later it will get sticky and hard to clean.

A RECIPE FOR FRIDAY NIGHT SPAGHETTI

I am sure you can figure it out from here.

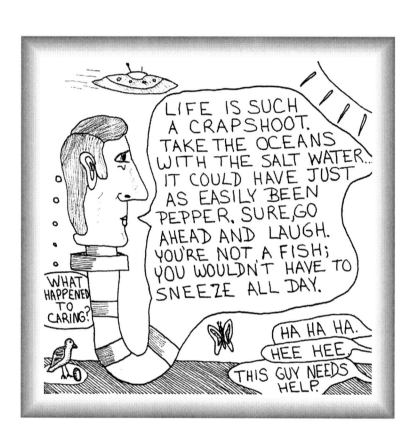

CHAPTER TWELVE

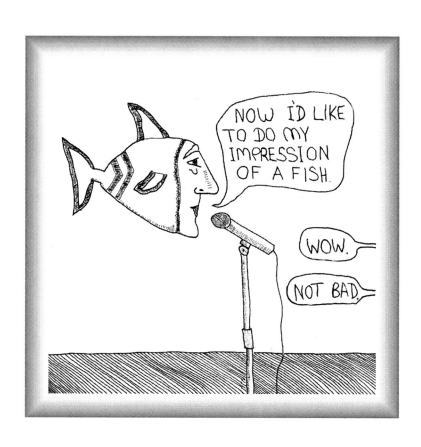

60

SUGGESTIONS

The Bowl Suggestion

I used to use a big bowl when I ate spaghetti
and I filled it to the brim
and I always went back for seconds,
even thirds.
Now I use a smaller bowl
and I don't fill it up as much
and I don't go back for seconds,
except during the holidays.
Thirds are history.

SUGGESTIONS

The Pass-The-Time Suggestion

Sometimes I would eat between things I had to do,
you know, on a break from work or to pass the time.
I am talking about potato chips, popcorn, a candy bar,
a peanut butter and jelly sandwich, a bowl of vanilla ice cream,
a quick burger and fries at a fast food place.
It is not a good idea to do this.
The part in Chapter One about eating less is
definitely talking about this kind of eating.

SUGGESTIONS

The Sink-Repair Suggestion

Open the doors under the kitchen sink,
take out all the stuff inside the cabinet,
lie down on your back,
shove yourself inside the cabinet under the sink,
reach up and tighten the nut underneath one of the sink faucets.
If your belly twitches and you are uncomfortable,
you need to read Chapter Two... maybe Chapter One as well.

SUGGESTIONS

The Frozen-Juice Suggestion
When you make lemonade
from the frozen concentrated kind,
if it says to add three cans of water, add five instead.
You get more juice and it is not so sweet.

SUGGESTIONS

The Read-The-Label Suggestion

Besides having a lot of salt in food these days,
there is a lot of other stuff that is not always good for you.
If you read the label on the can or box or package,
you will see what is in the food.
If you do not understand all of it, ask a teenager because
they teach them about labels in Health class.

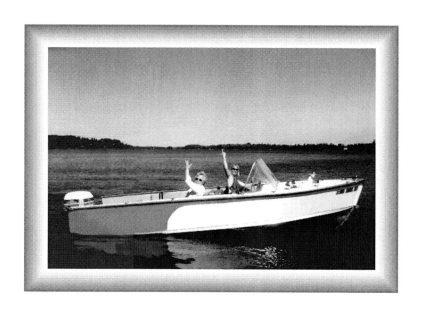

CHAPTER THIRTEEN

This scientific-looking chart
shows the probability of feeling better
if you lose weight and get in shape.

SCIENTIFIC·LOOKING CHART

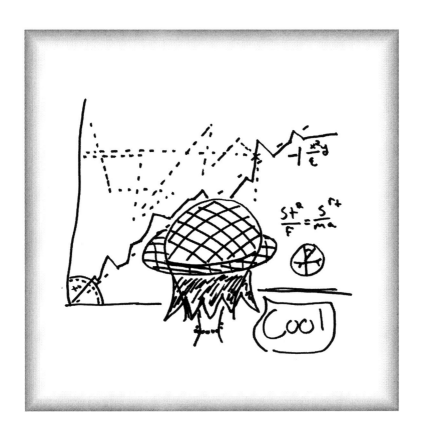

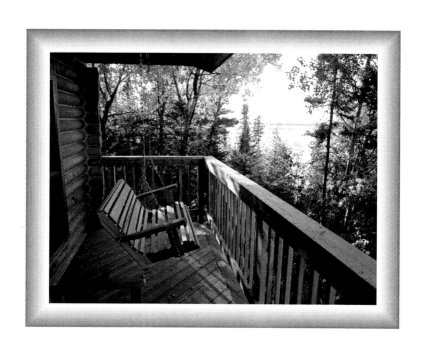

BONUS NOTICE

My big sister said I should put something in the book about
getting enough rest and remembering to relax.

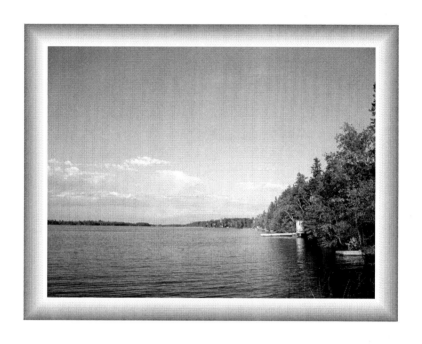

CHAPTER FOURTEEN

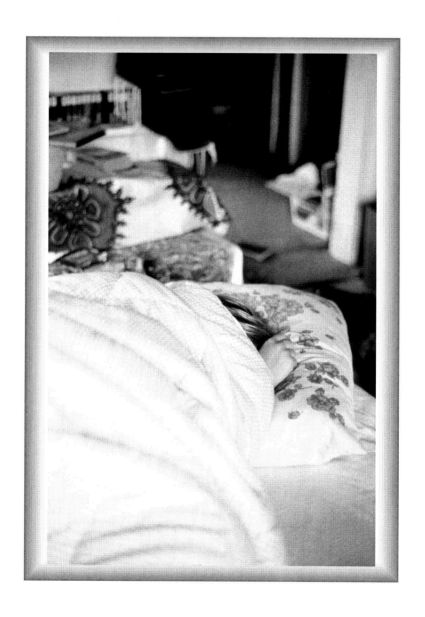

It is important to get enough rest and remember to relax.

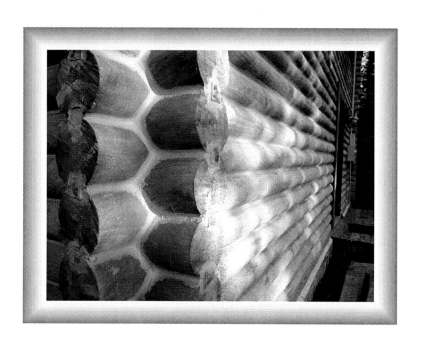

CHAPTER FIFTEEN

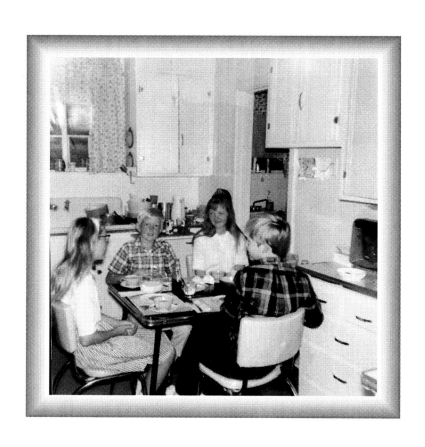

My cousin, who is a teacher, told me
that the book should have a really good ending.

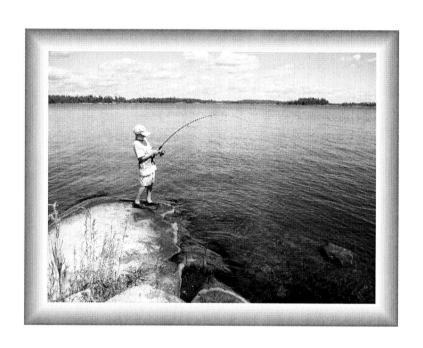

CHAPTER SIXTEEN

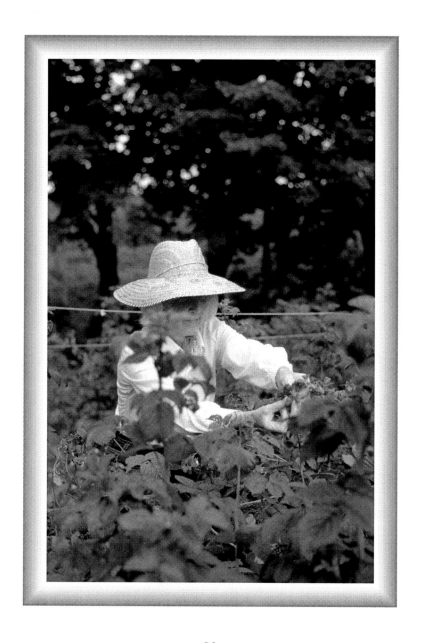

We're getting close to the end,
so if there is anything else that you think should be in this book,
you know, about losing weight and getting in shape,
jot it down here.

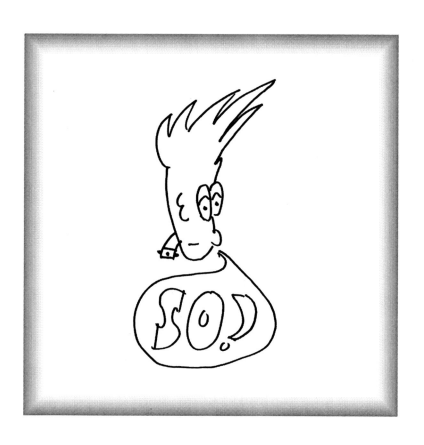

CHAPTER
SEVENTEEN

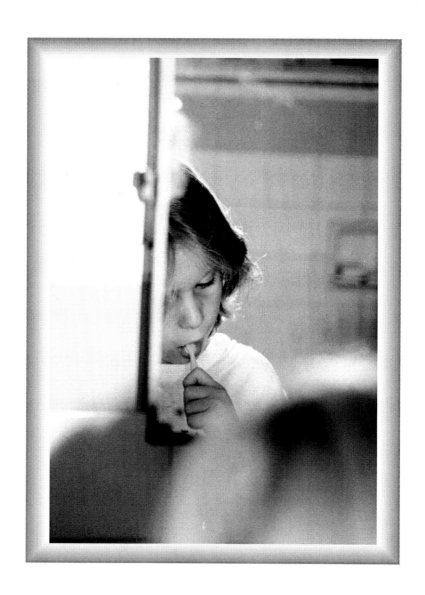

OK then, nothing else to add so that pretty much wraps it up.
Next is the big conclusion.

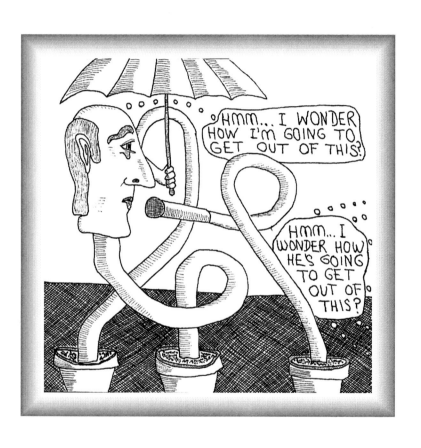

CONCLUSION

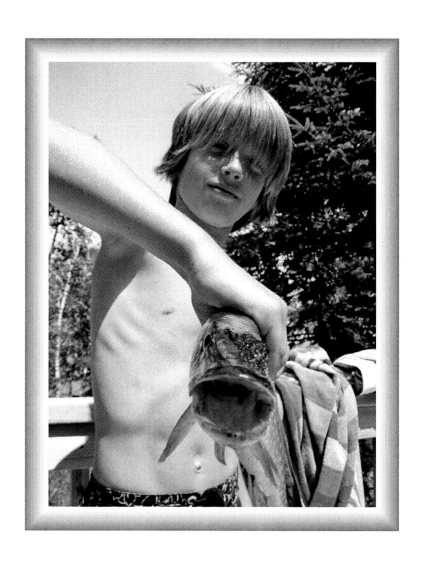

The most important part of this book is
Chapter One and Chapter Two.

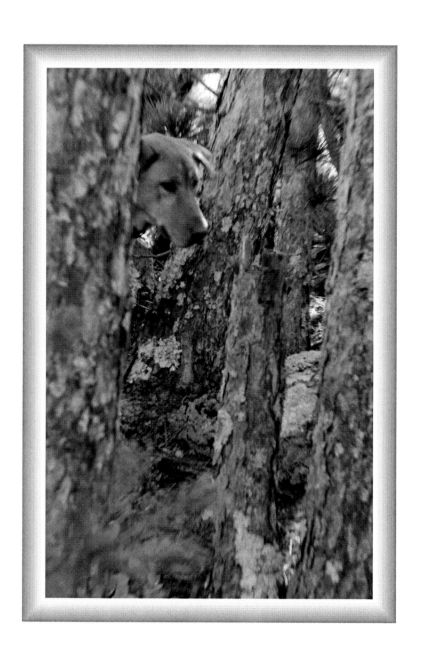

LAST NOTICE

I just remembered that the other morning
while we were having coffee,
my wife told me that good books
(I think she might have said "serious books")
have an appendix section after the conclusion.
I told her I couldn't do that because
I already had mine taken out, ha ha.

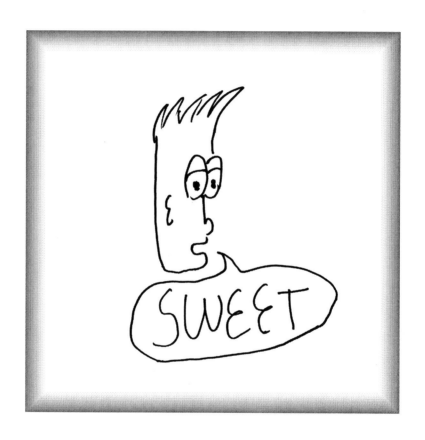

APPENDIX A

Illustrations and Photographs
by
An A, Three Bs, and a D

Our Next Comedian	*xii	Say What?	**46
Good Spaghetti	xiv	Wastage	**48
Road	2	Sunset Ritual	50
Jump	4	Pepper Water	*58
Pump House	6	Fish Impression	*60
Bakery	8	Queen Mary	66
Sniffing	10	Chart	**69
Quite a Town	*12	The Log Swing	70
Eyes	14	Lake to the East	72
Hilwa on the Dock	16	Sleep	74
Icicle	18	Log Corner	76
Shoveling Snow	20	The Kitchen Table	78
Cap and Plaid	22	Snag	80
Breakfast Table	24	Raspberries	82
Leaves	26	So!	**84
Hand in the Heartland	28	Brushing Teeth	86
Dusk Fishing	30	I Wonder	*88
Eagle	32	Keeper	90
Mowing	34	Of the North	92
Dishes	36	Sweet	**94
Fine Ladies	*38	Middle School	96
Poplar and Pine	40	School Morning	98
Schooled	**42	Nose	100
Affects Me How?	**44	Dock Portrait	103

* illustration by Bill McDonald
** illustration by Brian McDonald
photographs by family and friends

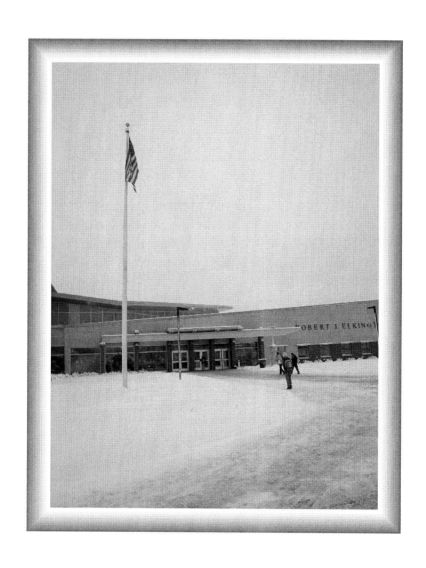

APPENDIX B

Here is a folk story I like. You might have already heard it.

∎∎∎∎

There was a farmer working in his field when a traveler walked up.
He asked the farmer,
"What sort of folk live in the town up ahead?"
The farmer replied,
"What sort of people live in the town where you came from?"
The traveler responded,
"They are hard-working, honest, good people."
"Oh," the farmer said,
"that's the sort of people you will find here as well."
"Well, thank you sir," said the traveler and headed into town.

A few days later another traveler came along
and yelled to the farmer,
"What sort of people live in this town?"
The farmer replied,
"What sort of people live in the town where you came from?"
The traveler grumbled,
"Bad, lazy, good-for-nothings. I'm glad I moved away."
"Hmm," replied the old farmer,
"I'm afraid you'll find the folks in this town
to be just about the same."
The traveler shook his head and continued on his way.

∎∎∎∎

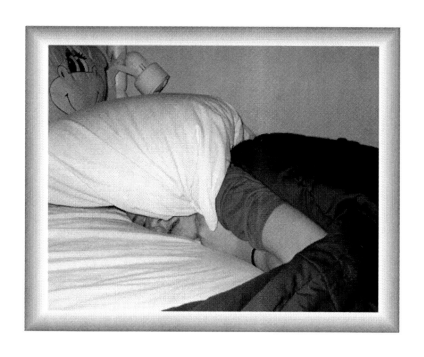

APPENDIX C

My big sister, the one who said I should have something
in the book about getting enough rest and remembering to relax,
wrote the following and told me I better include it
and pretend that I wrote it.

⊟⊟⊟⊟

"I want to express my deep appreciation to my beloved sister
who encouraged me to pursue my dream.
Not only was she there for me emotionally
as I labored over this project
but she also put in hours of research
and read my manuscript in countless drafts.
Any mistakes are mine and do not reflect
on her tireless pursuit of perfection."
- Sven Olsen

⊟⊟⊟⊟

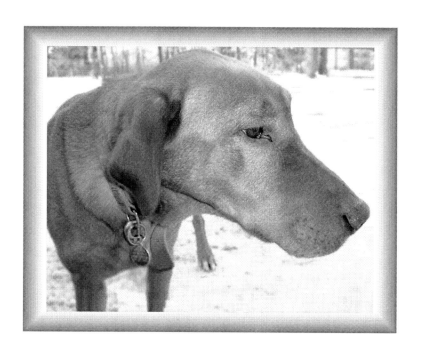

THE END

That's my wife and me with our dog.

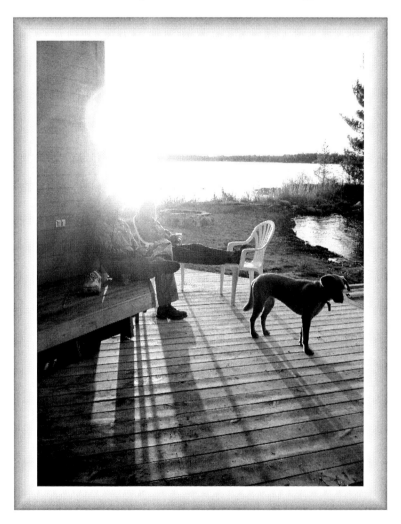

ABOUT THE AUTHOR

Not much is known about Sven Olsen and that seems to work well with him. When asked to provide some biographical details for this section of the book, Sven referred all our inquiries to his dog, Hilwa.

"Sven is a pretty quiet and private kind of guy," says David McDonald of DMcD Productions, Inc., the publisher of "OH FOR SMART".

McDonald says that it was a chance meeting at the YMCA in Grand Rapids, Minnesota where he happened to hear about Sven's pretty good way to lose weight and get in shape.

"We were both doing some stretching and I complimented Sven on his "OH FOR SMART" t-shirt and asked what sizes they came in. He said the usual sizes and then, quite unlike him, he just started telling me all about how he had to switch from a large to an extra large t-shirt a while back. Then one morning he put on an extra large t-shirt and it felt a little tight. So he had a cup of coffee and pretty much put together the whole "OH FOR SMART" routine right then and there. Pretty amazing, eh?"

For what little information there is about Sven, please go to
www.ohforsmart.com